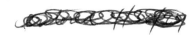

The JUICE ADVANTAGE

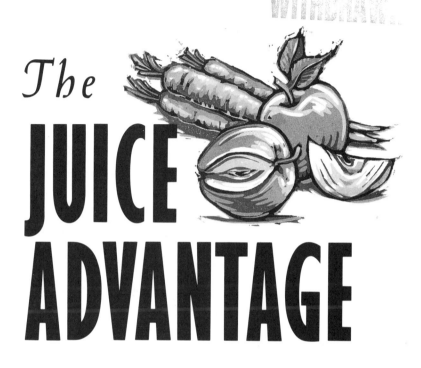

JAY KORDICH

with

MICHAEL T. MURRAY, N.D.

D1550408

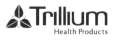
Health Products

Seattle, Washington

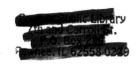

Important
Please Read

The information in this book is intended to increase your knowledge of fresh fruit and vegetable juicing. By no means is it intended to diagnose or treat an individual's health problems or ailments. The information given is not medical advice nor is it presented as medical advice. Before starting any type of diet or medical treatment, you should consult your own health care practitioner.

ISBN 0-9630948-1-5

Library of Congress Catalog Card Number 92-64381

Printed in the United States of America.

Cover illustrations by Kris Wiltse.

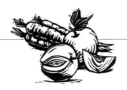

Contents

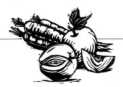

Introduction

The quality of your life begins with the quality of the foods that sustain it, and the surest path to a healthier, more energetic, and disease-free lifestyle begins with a diet rich in fresh fruit and vegetable juices. Fresh juices provide the proteins, enzymes, carbohydrates, essential fatty acids, vitamins and minerals that are vital to the health of your body.

The advantages of increased energy, strengthened immunity from illness and disease, strong bones and the glowing complexion that is the evidence of great health can all be yours when fresh fruit and vegetable juices form a substantial part of your daily diet. It is a well known fact that the Surgeon General, the Secretary of Health and Human Services, the National Cancer Institute and many others are all saying the same thing: *"Eat more fresh fruits and vegetables!"* Juicing provides the nutritional advantages of fruits and vegetables in a concentrated form that is easily absorbed by the body, and is the most enjoyable and efficient way to increase your consumption of these life-giving foods.

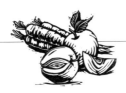

I

What Do Americans Eat?

The so-called standard American diet (SAD) does not provide adequate levels of fruits and vegetables. Instead, most Americans focus on refined foods high in calories, sugar, fat and cholesterol. Instead of eating life-giving foods, Americans are filling up on cheeseburgers, french fries, Twinkies and chocolate chip cookies, and washing them down with artificially colored and flavored fruit drinks or colas. It is a "SAD" fact that the three leading causes of death in the U.S. (heart disease, cancer and strokes) are diet related, and that over one-third of our adult population is overweight.

It has been estimated that in one year, the average American consumes 100 pounds of refined sugar and 55 pounds of fats and oils in the form of:

- 300 cans of soda pop
- 200 sticks of gum
- 18 pounds of candy
- 5 pounds of potato chips

- 7 pounds of corn chips, popcorn and pretzels
- 63 dozen donuts and pastries
- 50 pounds of cakes and cookies
- 20 gallons of ice cream

On top of this, nearly one-third of our adult population smokes and at least 10 percent are alcoholics. Then consider the health effects of the over 4 billion pounds of food additives, pesticides and herbicides added to our foods each year. Is it any wonder we are sick? Is it any wonder that as a nation we rank lower in life expectancy than sixteen other industrial nations, despite the fact that we spend more money on health care (a projected $813 billion for 1992) than any nation in the world?

The Role of Diet in Disease Prevention

An extensive body of knowledge has clearly established the link between the standard American diet (high fat, high sugar, low fiber) and the development of the primary "diseases of civilization" (heart disease, several types of cancers, strokes, high blood pressure, diabetes, gallstones, arthritis and more).[1] How can we prevent disease? By adopting a healthy diet and lifestyle. In fact, because these diseases are found much less frequently in vegetarians, it has been suggested that a vegetarian diet be the model for risk reduction of these major killers.[2-4]

At the bare minimum, we should follow the seven dietary recommendations given by the American Cancer Society, which are designed to significantly reduce the risk for cancer.[5] These recommendations are as follows:

- Avoid obesity.
- Reduce total fat intake to less than 30 percent of total calories.
- Eat more high-fiber foods, such as whole grain cereals, legumes, fruits and vegetables.
- Emphasize fruits and vegetables for their carotene and

Estimated Total Deaths and % of Total Deaths for the 10 Leading Causes of Death: United States, 1987

Rank	Cause of Death	Number	% of Total Deaths
1	**Heart diseases**	**759,400**	**35.7**
2	**Cancers**	**476,700**	**22.4**
3	**Strokes**	**148,700**	**7.0**
4	Unintentional injuries	92,500	4.4
5	Chronic obstructive lung disease	78,000	3.7
6	Pneumonia & influenza	68,600	3.2
7	**Diabetes mellitus**	**37,800**	**1.8**
8	Suicide	29,600	1.4
9	Chronic liver disease & cirrhosis	26,000	1.2
10	**Atherosclerosis**	**23,100**	**1.1**
	All Causes	**2,125,100**	**100.0**

Causes of death in which diet plays a part are in bold.

From the Surgeon General's report on Nutrition and Health.
Source: National Center for Health Statistics, *Monthly Vital Statistics Report,* vol. 37, no. 1, April 25, 1988.

vitamin C content.
- Include cruciferous vegetables such as cabbage, broccoli, Brussels sprouts and cauliflower in the diet for their anti-cancer compounds.
- Be moderate in the consumption of alcoholic beverages.
- Be moderate in the consumption of salt-cured, smoked and nitrite-cured foods.

Where does juicing figure into these recommendations? Quite simply, without juicing it is extremely difficult to get the amount of nutrition we need to reduce our risks for not only cancer, but heart disease and strokes. For example, recent studies indicate that to effectively reduce the risk of many cancers we would need to eat in a day the amount of beta-carotene equivalent to about two to three pounds of fresh carrots (roughly six large carrots).[6-10] To thoroughly chew one carrot takes approximately 10–15 minutes, so to eat six could take 1–1½ hours per day. Most Americans simply do not have the desire, nor the time, to do this. On the other hand, one 16-ounce glass of carrot juice will provide this same carotene equivalent. Juicing provides a quick, easy and effective way to meet your daily quota of carotenes and other valuable cancer-fighting nutrients.

Juicing and Weight Control

Many Americans are overfed but undernourished. Estimates are that up to 50 percent of our adult population is overweight. Juicing helps reset the body's appetite control center by providing the high quality nutrition it needs. This is vitally important at all times, but is especially important during weight loss. If the body is not fed, it feels that it is starving. As a result, metabolism will slow down. This means less fat will be burned. Juicing is an excellent way to supply key nutrients to the body in a fresh, raw and natural way.

Diets containing a high percentage of uncooked foods are significantly associated with weight loss and the lowering of blood pressure in overweight individuals.[11] Researchers seeking to determine why raw food diets produce these effects have made the following conclusions:

A raw food diet is much more satisfying to the appetite. Cooking can cause the loss of up to 97 percent of water-soluble vitamins (B vitamins and vitamin C) and up to 40 percent of fat-soluble vitamins (A, D, E and K). Since uncooked foods such as juices contain more vitamins and other nutrients, they are more satisfying to the body. The result is reduced calorie intake and weight loss in obese individuals.

The blood pressure lowering effect of raw foods is most likely due to healthier food choices, fiber and potassium. However, the effect of cooking the food cannot be ruled out. When patients are switched from a raw food diet to a cooked diet (without a change in calorie or sodium content), there is a rapid increase of blood pressure back to pre-study levels.

A diet in which an average of 60 percent of calories ingested come from raw foods reduces stress on the body. Specifically, the presence of enzymes in raw foods, the reduced allergenicity of raw foods, and the effects of raw foods on our gut-bacteria ecosystem are thought to be much more healthful than the effects of cooked foods.

Juicing is a phenomenal way to reach the goal of ingesting 60 percent of total calories from raw foods. More and more experts are making this recommendation to encourage people to improve the nutritional quality of their diets. As a bonus, juicing helps the body's digestive process and allows for quick absorption of high quality nutrition. The result? Increased energy levels. This is one of the greatest advantages of utilizing fresh juice in a weight-loss plan.

Some juices are better than others for promoting weight loss. The most beneficial juices for promoting weight loss are those that are dense in nutrients, but low in calories. The following are the most nutrient-dense fruits and vegetables suitable for juicing:

1. Bell peppers
2. Parsley
3. Kale
4. Broccoli
5. Spinach
6. Celery
7. Brussels sprouts
8. Cauliflower

9. Carrots
10. Cabbage
11. Beets
12. Pineapple
13. Cantaloupe
14. Watermelon
15. Tomatoes
16. Apple
17. Strawberries
18. Pears
19. Oranges
20. Grapes

The first eight vegetables listed are not only dense in nutrients, they are quite powerful. Mixing them with carrot, apple or tomato juice will make them much more palatable. Notice that the fruits are further down on the scale than the vegetables. Although fruits are full of valuable nutrients, they contain more natural sugars than vegetables. This means they are higher in calories, so they should be used sparingly.

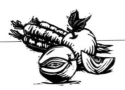

2
What's In Juice?

Fresh fruit and vegetable juice is a source of natural water and provides the body with easily absorbed protein, carbohydrate, essential fatty acids, vitamins and minerals. In addition, fresh juice provides enzymes, pigments like carotenes, chlorophyll and flavonoids, and numerous accessory food components known as anutrients.

Enzymes are protein molecules that are responsible for speeding up chemical reactions. Enzymes are what make plants alive and give us life as well. Plant pigments, especially carotenes and flavonoids, are remarkable in their ability to protect our cells from damage. The accessory components, or anutrients, found in fresh juice can help fight cancer and promote health.

Water
Vital for Optimal Performance

It's appropriate to first point out that fresh juice provides natural water. Water is the most plentiful substance in our bodies. Each day we require an intake of over two quarts of water to function optimally. About one quart each day is provided in the foods that we eat. This means that we need to drink at least one quart of liquids each day to maintain good water balance. More is needed in warmer climates or for physically active people.

There is currently a great concern over our water supply. It is becoming increasingly difficult to find pure water. Most of our water supply is full of chemicals including not only chlorine and fluoride, which are routinely added, but a wide range of toxic organic compounds and chemicals such as PCBs, pesticide residues, nitrates and heavy metals like lead, mercury and cadmium.[12]

Drinking fresh fruit and vegetable juice (especially if derived from organic produce) is a fantastic way to give your body the natural pure water it desires. Water is vital to our health. It constitutes over 60 percent of our body weight. Over two-thirds of the body's water content is found inside the cells. The rest is found coursing through our bodies carrying vital nutrients and blood cells. In addition, water functions in chemical reactions, serves as a lubricant in our joints, aids in maintaining body temperature, and serves as an insulator and shock absorber in body compartments.

Not drinking enough liquids or eating enough high water-content foods puts a great deal of stress on the body. Kidney function is likely to be affected, gallstones and kidney stones are likely to form, and immune function will be impaired. It is clear that water is one of our most critical nutrients, and juicing is a fantastic way to meet body water requirements.

Protein
Essential to Good Health

After water, protein is the next most plentiful component in our bodies. The body manufactures proteins to make up hair, muscles, nails, tendons, ligaments and other body structures. Proteins also function as enzymes, hormones and important components to other cells such as our genes. Adequate protein intake is essential to good health. In fact, advertisers for the meat and dairy industry have spent a great deal of money educating us about the importance of protein. They have done such a good job that most Americans consume far greater amounts of protein than the body actually requires. The recommended daily allowance for protein is 44 grams for the average woman and 56 grams for the average man, or approximately 8–9 percent of total daily calories. Most Americans consume almost twice this amount.

Proteins are composed of individual building blocks known as amino acids. The human body can manufacture most of the amino acids required for making body proteins. However, there are nine amino acids that the body cannot manufacture. These are termed "essential" amino acids. The essential amino acids required from our dietary intake are arginine, histidine, isoleucine, lysine, methionine, phenylalanine, threonine, tryptophan and valine. The quality of a protein source is based on its levels of these essential amino acids, along with its digestibility and its ability to be utilized by the body.

A complete protein source is one that provides all of the nine essential amino acids in adequate amounts. Animal products—meat, fish, dairy and poultry—are examples of complete proteins. Plant foods, especially grains and legumes (beans), often lack one or more of the essential amino acids, but become complete when they are combined. For example, combining grains with legumes results in a complete protein, as the two protein sources complement each other. By consuming a varied diet of grains, legumes, fruits and vegetables, and by maintaining a sufficient calorie content, a person is almost assured of getting complete proteins.

Fresh fruits and vegetables often contain the full complement of amino acids. But because fruits and vegetables contain protein in lower quantities, they are generally considered poor protein sources. However, as previously mentioned, the nutritional qualities of fruits and vegetables become concentrated in their juice form, making juices an excellent source of easily absorbed amino acids and proteins. For example, sixteen ounces of carrot juice (the equivalent of two to three pounds of fresh raw carrots) will provide nearly 5 grams

Percentage of Calories as Protein

Legumes		Grains	
Soybean sprouts	54%	Wheat germ	31%
Mung bean sprouts	43%	Rye	20%
Soybean curd (tofu)	43%	Wheat, hard red	17%
Soyflour	35%	Wild rice	16%
Soy sauce	33%	Buckwheat	15%
Broad beans	32%	Oatmeal	15%
Lentils	29%	Millet	12%
Split peas	28%	Barley	11%
Kidney beans	26%	Brown rice	8%
Navy beans	26%		
Lima beans	26%	**Nuts and Seeds**	
Garbanzo beans	23%	Pumpkin seeds	21%
		Peanuts	18%
Vegetables		Sunflower seeds	17%
Spinach	49%	Walnuts, black	13%
Kale	45%	Sesame seeds	13%
Broccoli	45%	Almonds	12%
Brussels sprouts	44%	Cashews	12%
Turnip greens	43%	Filberts	8%
Collard greens	43%		
Cauliflower	40%	**Fruits**	
Mushrooms	38%	Lemons	16%
Parsley	34%	Honeydew melon	10%
Lettuce	34%	Cantaloupe	9%
Green peas	30%	Strawberries	8%
Zucchini	28%	Oranges	8%
Green beans	26%	Blackberries	8%
Cucumbers	24%	Cherries	8%
Green peppers	22%	Grapes	8%
Artichokes	22%	Watermelon	8%
Cabbage	22%	Tangerines	7%
Celery	21%	Papayas	6%
Eggplant	21%	Peaches	6%
Tomatoes	18%	Pears	5%
Onions	16%	Bananas	5%
Beets	15%	Grapefruit	5%
Pumpkin	12%	Pineapple	3%
Potatoes	11%	Apples	1%

Source: "Nutritive Value of American Foods in Common Units,"
U.S.D.A. Agriculture Handbook No. 456

of protein. Obviously, fresh juice should not be relied upon to meet all of your body's protein needs. You will need other protein sources as well, such as grains and legumes. Or, add a protein supplement to your juice.

Carbohydrates
Provide Energy for the Body

Carbohydrates provide us with the energy we need for bodily functions. There are two groups of carbohydrates, simple and complex. Simple carbohydrates, or sugars, are quickly absorbed by the body for a ready source of energy. The assortment of natural simple sugars in fruits and vegetables have an advantage over sucrose (white sugar) and other refined sugars in that they are balanced by a wide range of nutrients that aid in the utilization of the sugars. Problems with carbohydrates begin when they are refined and stripped of these nutrients. Virtually all of the vitamin content has been removed from white sugar, white breads and pastries, and many breakfast cereals. When high sugar foods are eaten alone, the blood sugar level rises quickly, producing a strain on blood sugar control. Too much of any simple sugar, including the sugars found in fruit and vegetable juices, can be harmful—especially if you are hypoglycemic, diabetic or prone to candida infection. Since fruit juices are higher in sugars than vegetable juices, their use should be limited. Sources of refined sugar should be limited even more. Read food labels carefully for clues on sugar content. If the words sucrose, glucose, maltose, lactose, fructose, corn syrup, or white grape juice concentrate appear on the label, extra sugar has been added.

Complex carbohydrates, or starches, are composed of many sugars (polysaccharides) joined together by chemical bonds. The body breaks down complex carbohydrates into simple sugars gradually, which leads to better blood sugar control. More and more research is indicating that complex carbohydrates should form a major part of the diet. Vegetables, legumes and grains are excellent sources of complex carbohydrates.

17

Fats and Oils
Important Cellular Components

There is very little fat in fresh fruit or vegetable juices, but the fats that *are* contained in them are essential to human health. The essential fatty acids, linoleic acids and linolenic acids provided by fruits and vegetables function in our bodies as components of nerve cells, cellular membranes and hormone-like substances. Fats also provide the body with energy.

Animal fats are typically solid at room temperature and are referred to as saturated fats, while vegetable fats are liquid at room temperature and are referred to as unsaturated fats or oils. There is a great deal of research linking a diet high in saturated fat to numerous cancers, heart disease and strokes. Both the American Cancer Society and the American Heart Association have recommended a diet containing less than 30 percent of calories as fat. Looking at the chart opposite it is obvious that the easiest way for most people to achieve this goal is to eat fewer animal products and more plant foods.

Vitamins
Essential for Life

Vitamins function along with enzymes in the chemical reactions necessary for human bodily function, including energy production. Together, vitamins and enzymes work together to act as catalysts in speeding up the making or breaking of chemical bonds that join molecules together. For example, vitamin C functions in the manufacture of collagen, the main protein substance of the human body. Specifically, vitamin C is involved in joining a portion of the water molecule to the amino acid proline to form hydroxyproline. The result is a very stable collagen structure. Since collagen is such an important protein for the structures that hold our body together (like connective tissue, cartilage and tendons), vitamin C is vital for wound repair, healthy gums and the prevention of easy bruising.

Percentage of Calories as Fat

Eggs & Dairy Products

Butter	100%
Cream, light whipping	92%
Cream cheese	90%
Egg yolks	80%
Half-and-half	79%
Cheddar cheese	71%
Swiss cheese	66%
Eggs, whole	65%
Cow's milk	49%
Yogurt, plain	49%
Ice cream, regular	48%
Cottage cheese	35%
Lowfat (2%) milk/yogurt	31%

Meats

Sirloin steak*	83%
Pork sausage	83%
T-bone steak*	82%
Porterhouse steak*	82%
Bologna	81%
Spareribs	80%
Frankfurters	80%
Lamb rib chops*	79%
Salami	76%
Rump roast*	71%
Ham*	69%
Ground beef, fairly lean	64%
Veal Breast*	64%
Leg of lamb	61%
Round steak*	61%
Chicken, dark meat[+]	56%
Chuck steak, lean only	50%
Turkey, dk. meat w/skin	47%
Chicken, light meat[+]	44%

Fruits

Grapes	11%
Strawberries	11%
Apples	8%
Blueberries	7%
Lemons	7%
Pears	5%
Apricots	4%
Oranges	4%
Bananas	4%
Cantaloupe	3%
Pineapple	3%
Grapefruit	2%
Papayas	2%
Peaches	2%
Prunes	1%

Vegetables

Mustard greens	13%
Kale	13%
Beet greens	12%
Lettuce	12%
Turnip greens	11%
Cabbage	7%
Cauliflower	7%
Green beans	6%
Celery	6%
Cucumbers	6%
Turnips	6%
Zucchini	6%
Carrots	4%
Green peas	4%
Beets	2%
Potatoes	1%

* Lean, with fat. + With skin, roasted.

Source: "Nutritive Value of American Foods in Common Units,"
U.S.D.A. Agriculture Handbook No. 456

There are fifteen different known vitamins, each with its own special role to play. The vitamins are classified into two groups: fat-soluble (A, D, E and K) and water-soluble (the B vitamins and vitamin C). Vitamins are essential to good health; without them key body processes would halt. Low levels of vitamins and minerals within our bodies may be preventing many of us from achieving optimal health.

Juicing allows for concentration of nutrition and gives us key nutrients in their most natural form. This makes fresh fruit and vegetables juice a rich source of water-soluble vitamins and some fat-soluble vitamins (provitamin A carotenes and vitamin K). Fresh fruit or vegetable juice is more nutritious than cooked fruits or vegetables, as cooking destroys many of the B vitamins and vitamin C.

While most people think of fruits as the best source of vitamin C, vegetables also contain high levels, especially broccoli, peppers, potatoes and Brussels sprouts. For the B vitamins (except vitamin B_{12}), your best sources are grains and green leafy vegetables like spinach, kale, parsley and broccoli.[13,14]

One vitamin that is often neglected is vitamin K. Vitamin K_1, the form of vitamin K that is found in green leafy vegetables, has a role in converting inactive osteocalcin to its active form. Osteocalcin is the major noncollagen protein found in our bones. Vitamin K_1 is necessary for allowing the osteocalcin molecule to bind the calcium and hold it into place within the bone.

A deficiency of vitamin K_1 leads to impaired mineralization of the bone due to inadequate osteocalcin levels. Very low blood levels of vitamin K_1 have been found in patients with fractures due to osteoporosis.[15,16] The severity of the fracture strongly correlated with the level of circulating vitamin K_1: the lower the level of vitamin K_1, the greater the severity of the fracture.

Vitamin K_1 is found in green leafy vegetables and may be one of the protective factors of a vegetarian diet against osteoporosis. Juices are an excellent source of naturally occurring vitamin K_1.

Vitamin C Content of Selected Foods

Milligrams (mg) per 100 grams edible portion (100 grams = 3.5 oz.)

Acerola	1,300	Liver, calf	36
Peppers, red chili	369	Turnips	36
Guavas	242	Mangoes	35
Peppers, red sweet	190	Asparagus	33
Kale leaves	186	Cantaloupe	33
Parsley	172	Swiss chard	32
Collard greens	152	Green onions	32
Turnip greens	139	Liver, beef	31
Peppers, green sweet	128	Okra	31
Broccoli	113	Tangerines	31
Brussels sprouts	102	New Zealand spinach	30
Mustard greens	97	Oysters	30
Watercress	79	Lima beans, young	29
Cauliflower	78	Black-eyed peas	29
Persimmons	66	Soybeans	29
Cabbage, red	61	Green peas	27
Strawberries	59	Radishes	26
Papayas	56	Raspberries	25
Spinach	51	Chinese cabbage	25
Oranges & juice	50	Yellow summer squash	25
Cabbage	47	Loganberries	24
Lemon juice	46	Honeydew melon	23
Grapefruit & juice	38	Tomatoes	23
Elderberries	36	Liver, pork	23

Source: "Nutritive Value of American Foods in Common Units,"
U.S.D.A Agriculture Handbook No. 456

Minerals
For Blood, Bone and Cell Functions

There are twenty-two different minerals important to human nutrition. Minerals function with vitamins as components of enzymes. Minerals are also needed for proper composition of bone and blood, and for the maintenance of normal cell function. The minerals are classified into two categories: major and minor. The major minerals include calcium, phosphorus, potassium, sodium, chloride, magnesium and sulfur. The minor (trace) minerals include iron, iodine, zinc, chromium, vanadium, silicon, selenium, copper, fluoride, cobalt, molybdenum, manganese, tin, boron and nickel.

Because plants incorporate minerals from the soil into their own tissues, fruits and vegetables are excellent sources for many minerals. The minerals, as they are found in the earth, are inorganic—lifeless. In plants, however, most minerals are complexed with organic molecules. This usually means better mineral absorption. Juicing is thought to provide even better mineral absorption compared to the intact fruit or vegetable because juicing liberates the minerals into a highly bio-available medium. The green leafy vegetables are the best source for many minerals, especially calcium.[13]

In addition to vitamin K_1, the high levels of many minerals found in plant foods may also be responsible for the protective effect of a vegetarian diet against osteoporosis. A trace mineral gaining recent attention as a protective factor against osteoporosis is boron. Boron has been shown to have a positive effect on calcium and active estrogen levels in postmenopausal women, the group at highest risk for developing osteoporosis. In one study, supplementing the diet of postmenopausal women with 3 mg of boron per day reduced urinary calcium excretion by 44 percent and dramatically increased the levels of 17-beta-estradiol, the most biologically active estrogen.[17] It appears boron is required to activate certain hormones including estrogen and vitamin D. Since fruits and vegetables are the main dietary sources of boron, diets low in these foods may be deficient in boron. The high boron content of a vegetarian diet may be another protective factor against osteoporosis.

22

Calcium Content of Selected Foods

Milligrams (mg) per 100 grams edible portion (100 grams = 3.5 oz.)

Kelp	1093	Globe artichokes	51
Cheddar cheese	750	Dried prunes	51
Carob flour	352	Pumpkin/squash seeds	51
Dulse	296	Cooked dry beans	50
Collard greens	250	Common cabbage	49
Kale	249	Soybean sprouts	48
Turnip greens	246	Hard winter wheat	46
Almonds	234	Oranges	41
Brewer's yeast	210	Celery	41
Parsley	203	Cashews	38
Dandelion greens	187	Rye grain	38
Brazil nuts	186	Carrots	37
Watercress	151	Barley	34
Goat milk	129	Sweet potatoes	32
Tofu	128	Brown rice	32
Dried figs	126	Garlic	29
Buttermilk	121	Summer squash	28
Sunflower seeds	120	Onions	27
Yogurt	120	Lemons	26
Wheat bran	119	Fresh green peas	26
Whole milk	118	Cauliflower	25
Buckwheat, raw	114	Cucumber	25
Sesame seeds, hulled	110	Lentils, cooked	25
Ripe olives	106	Sweet cherries	22
Broccoli	103	Asparagus	22
English walnuts	99	Winter squash	22
Cottage cheese	94	Strawberries	21
Soybeans, cooked	73	Millet	20
Pecans	73	Pineapple	17
Wheat germ	72	Grapes	16
Peanuts	69	Beets	15
Miso	68	Cantaloupe	14
Romaine lettuce	68	Tomatoes	13
Dried apricots	67	Eggplant	12
Rutabagas	66	Chicken	12
Raisins	62	Avocados	10
Black currants	60	Beef	10
Dates	59	Banana	8
Green snap beans	56	Apple	7

Source: "Nutritive Value of American Foods in Common Units,"
U.S.D.A Agriculture Handbook No. 456

Potassium

Key to Blood Pressure Maintenance

One of the primary nutritional benefits of fresh juices is that they are very rich in potassium and very low in sodium.[13,14] The balance of sodium to potassium is extremely important to human health. Too much sodium in the diet can lead to disruption of this balance. Numerous studies have demonstrated that a low potassium, high sodium diet plays a major role in the development of cancer and cardiovascular disease (heart disease, high blood pressure and stroke).[18,19] Conversely, a diet high in potassium and low in sodium is protective against these diseases, and in the case of high blood pressure, it can be therapeutic.[19,20]

Excessive consumption of dietary sodium chloride (table salt), coupled with diminished dietary potassium, is a common cause of high blood pressure. Numerous studies have shown that sodium restriction alone does not improve blood pressure control in most people—it must be accompanied by a high potassium intake.[14,20] In our society only 5 percent of sodium intake comes from the natural ingredients in food. Prepared foods contribute 45 percent of our sodium intake, 45 percent is added in cooking, and another 5 percent is added as a condiment.

Most Americans have a potassium-to-sodium (K:Na) ratio of less than 1:2. This means most people ingest twice as much sodium as potassium. Researchers recommend a dietary potassium-to-sodium ratio of greater than 5:1 to maintain health. This is ten times higher than the average intake. However, even this may not be optimal. A natural diet rich in fruits and vegetables can produce a K:Na ratio greater than 100:1, as most fruits and vegetables have a K:Na ratio of at least 50:1.[20] For example, here are the average K:Na ratios for several common fresh fruits and vegetables:

- Carrots   75:1
- Potatoes   110:1
- Apples   90:1
- Bananas   440:1
- Oranges   260:1

Functions of Potassium

Potassium is one of the electrolytes—mineral salts that can conduct electricity when they are dissolved in water. Electrolytes are always found in pairs; a positive molecule like sodium or potassium is always accompanied by a negative molecule like chloride. Potassium, as a major electrolyte, functions in the maintenance of:

- Water balance and distribution
- Acid-base balance
- Muscle and nerve cell function
- Heart function
- Kidney and adrenal function

Over 95 percent of the potassium in the body is found within cells. In contrast, most of the sodium in the body is located outside cells in the blood and other fluids. How does this happen? Cells actually pump sodium out and potassium in via the "sodium-potassium pump." This pump is found in the membranes of all cells in the body. One of its most important functions is preventing the swelling of cells. If sodium is not pumped out, water accumulates within the cell, causing it to swell and ultimately burst.

The sodium-potassium pump also functions to maintain the electrical charge within the cell. This is particularly important to muscle and nerve cells. During nerve transmission and muscle contraction, potassium exits the cell and sodium enters, resulting in a change in electrical charge. This change is what causes a nerve impulse or muscle contraction. It is not surprising that a potassium deficiency affects muscles and nerves first.

Potassium deficiency

Potassium is essential for the conversion of blood sugar into glycogen—the storage form of blood sugar found in the muscles and liver. A potassium shortage results in lower levels of stored glycogen. Because glycogen is used by exercising muscles for energy, a potassium deficiency will produce great fatigue and muscle weakness. These are typically the first signs of potassium deficiency.

25

A potassium deficiency is characterized by mental confusion, irritability, weakness, heart disturbances and problems in nerve conduction and muscle contraction. Dietary potassium deficiency is typically caused by a diet low in fresh fruits and vegetables but high in sodium. It is more common to see dietary potassium deficiency in the elderly. Dietary potassium deficiency is less common than deficiency due to excessive fluid loss (sweating, diarrhea or urination) or the use of diuretics, laxatives, aspirin and other drugs.

The amount of potassium lost in sweat can be quite significant, especially if the exercise is prolonged in a warm environment. Athletes or people who regularly exercise have higher potassium needs. Because up to 3 grams of potassium can be lost in one day through sweating, a daily intake of at least 4 grams of potassium is recommended for athletic individuals.

How much potassium do we need?

The estimated safe and adequate daily dietary intake of potassium, as set by the Committee on Recommended Daily Allowances, is between 1.9 and 5.6 grams. If body potassium requirements are not being met through diet, supplementation is essential for good health. This is particularly true for the elderly and the athletic. Potassium salts are commonly prescribed by physicians in the dosage range of 1.5 to 3.0 grams per day. However, potassium salts can cause nausea, vomiting, diarrhea and ulcers. These effects are not seen when potassium levels are increased through the diet only. This highlights the advantages of using juices, foods or food-based potassium supplements to meet the human body's high potassium requirements. Most fruit and vegetable juices contain approximately 400 mg of potassium per 8-ounce cup.

While it is possible to get too much potassium, most people can handle any excess. The exceptions are people with kidney disease, who do not handle potassium in the normal way and are likely to experience heart disturbances and other consequences of potassium toxicity. Those with kidney disease should restrict their potassium intake and follow the dietary recommendations of their physician.

Potassium Content of Selected Foods

Milligrams (mg) per 100 grams edible portion (100 grams = 3.5 oz.)

Dulse	8,060	Cauliflower	295
Kelp	5,273	Watercress	282
Sunflower seeds	920	Asparagus	278
Wheat germ	827	Red cabbage	268
Almonds	773	Lettuce	264
Raisins	763	Cantaloupe	251
Parsley	727	Lentils, cooked	249
Brazil nuts	715	Tomatoes	244
Peanuts	674	Sweet potatoes	243
Dates	648	Papayas	234
Figs, dried	640	Eggplant	214
Avocados	604	Green peppers	213
Pecans	603	Beets	208
Yams	600	Peaches	202
Swiss chard	550	Summer squash	202
Soybeans, cooked	540	Oranges	200
Garlic	529	Raspberries	199
Spinach	470	Cherries	191
English walnuts	450	Strawberries	164
Millet	430	Grapefruit juice	162
Beans, cooked	416	Cucumbers	160
Mushrooms	414	Grapes	158
Potato with skin	407	Onions	157
Broccoli	382	Pineapple	146
Kale	378	Milk, whole	144
Bananas	370	Lemon juice	141
Meats	370	Pears	130
Winter squash	369	Eggs	129
Chicken	366	Apples	110
Carrots	341	Watermelon	100
Celery	341	Brown rice, cooked	70
Radishes	322		

Source: "Nutritive Value of American Foods in Common Units,"
U.S.D.A. Agriculture Handbook No. 456

Antioxidants
Protection Against Cellular Damage

Another key benefit of juicing is its ability to provide high levels of natural plant compounds that can protect against cellular damage. The cells of the human body are constantly under attack. The culprits? Free radicals and pro-oxidants. *Free radicals* are molecules that contain a highly reactive unpaired electron; *pro-oxidants* are molecules that can promote oxidative damage. These highly reactive molecules can bind to and destroy other cellular components. Free radical damage is a cause of aging, and is also linked to the development of cancer, heart disease, cataracts, Alzheimer's disease, arthritis, and virtually every other chronic degenerative disease.[21]

Sources of Free Radicals

Where do these sinister agents come from? Believe it or not, most of the free radicals zipping through our bodies are actually produced during normal metabolic processes like energy production, detoxification reactions and immune defense mechanisms. In fact, it is ironic that the major source of free radical damage in the body is the oxygen molecule—the molecule that gives us life is also the molecule that can do the most harm! Just as oxygen can rust iron, when toxic oxygen molecules are allowed to attack our cells, free radical or oxidative damage occurs.

Although the body's own generation of free radicals is important, the environment contributes greatly to the free radical load of an individual. Cigarette smoking, for example, greatly increases an individual's free radical load. Many of the harmful effects of smoking are related to the extremely high levels of free radicals being inhaled, depleting key antioxidant nutrients like vitamin C and beta-carotene.[22] Other external sources of free radicals include ionizing radiation, chemotherapeutic drugs, air pollutants, pesticides, anesthetics, aromatic hydrocarbons, fried food, solvents, alcohol, and formaldehyde. These compounds greatly stress the body's antioxidant mechanisms. Individuals exposed to these factors need additional nutritional support.[21]

How The Body Handles Free Radicals

Our cells protect against free radical and oxidative damage with the help of enzymes and antioxidants found in the plant foods we consume. These antioxidants include carotenes, flavonoids, vitamins C and E, and sulfur-containing compounds. Free radicals must be broken down by enzymes or be chemically neutralized before they react with cellular molecules. Examples of the free radical scavenging enzymes produced by the body are catalase, superoxide dismutase and glutathione peroxidase. Taking enzymes as an oral supplement is of limited value, as this has not been shown to increase enzyme tissue levels. However, ingesting antioxidant nutrients like manganese, sulfur-containing amino acids, carotenes, flavonoids and vitamin C, have been shown to increase tissue concentrations of the enzymes.[21-25,35]

The other way in which the cell can protect itself against free radical or oxidative damage is via chemical neutralization, antioxidants binding to or neutralizing the free radical or pro-oxidant. For example, the nutritional antioxidants (vitamin C, vitamin E, beta-carotene and selenium) block free radical damage by chemically reacting with the free radical or pro-oxidant to neutralize it. Ingesting rich sources of these compounds from fresh juices can increase tissue concentrations of these nutrients, thereby supporting normal cellular protective mechanisms.

Carotenes
Lower the Risk of Cancer

Carotenes, or carotenoids, represent the most widespread group of naturally occurring pigments in nature. They are a highly colored (red to yellow) group of fat-soluble compounds that function in plants to protect against damage produced during photosynthesis.[27] Carotenes are best known for their capacity to be converted into vitamin A, their antioxidant activity, and their correlation with the maximum life-span potential of humans, other primates and mammals.

29

Over 500 different carotenes have been characterized, but only about 30–50 are believed to have vitamin A activity. These are referred to as "provitamin A carotenes." The biological effects of a carotene have historically been based on its corresponding vitamin A activity. In fact, beta-carotene has been considered the most active of the carotenes because its provitamin A activity is higher than that of other carotenes. However, recent research suggests that these vitamin A activities have been overemphasized as there are other, nonvitamin A carotenes that exhibit far greater antioxidant and anticancer activities.[8,27]

The conversion of a provitamin A carotene into vitamin A is dependent on several factors: the level of vitamin A in the body, protein status, thyroid hormones, zinc and vitamin C. The conversion diminishes as carotene intake increases, and when serum vitamin A levels are adequate. If vitamin A levels are sufficient, the carotene is not converted to vitamin A. Instead it is delivered to body tissues for storage.[27]

Unlike vitamin A, which is stored primarily in the liver, unconverted carotenes are stored in fat cells, epithelial cells and other organs (the adrenals, testes and ovaries have the highest concentrations). Epithelial cells are found in the skin and the linings of our internal organs (including the respiratory tract, gastrointestinal tract and genitourinary tract).[8,27] Population studies have demonstrated a strong correlation between carotene intake and a variety of cancers involving epithelial tissues (such as lung, skin, uterine cervix and gastrointestinal tract tissues).[8-10,27] The higher the carotene intake, the lower the risk for cancer. Scientific studies are also showing that carotenes have antitumor and immune-enhancing activities.[27-30]

Cancer and aging share a number of common characteristics, including an association with free radical damage, which has led to the idea that the prevention of cancer should also promote longevity. There is some evidence to support this claim since it appears that tissue carotene content has a better correlation with maximum life-span potential (MLSP) of mammals, including humans, than any other factor that has been studied.[31] For example, the human MLSP of approximately 120 years correlates with serum carotene levels of 50–300 mcg/dl, while other primates such as the rhesus monkey have an MLSP of approximately 34 years correlating with serum carotene levels of 6–12 mcg/dl. The graph below demonstrates the relationships between the MLSP of several species and their corresponding carotenoid levels.

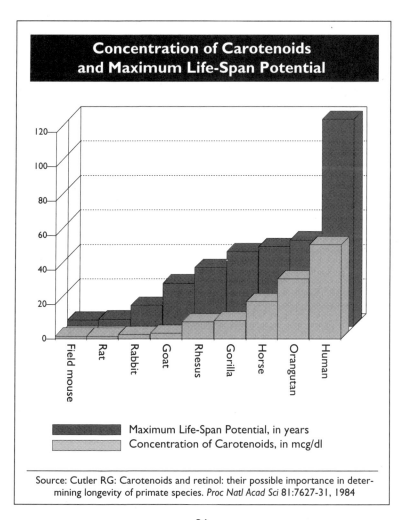

Concentration of Carotenoids and Maximum Life-Span Potential

Maximum Life-Span Potential, in years
Concentration of Carotenoids, in mcg/dl

Source: Cutler RG: Carotenoids and retinol: their possible importance in determining longevity of primate species. *Proc Natl Acad Sci* 81:7627-31, 1984

Since tissue carotenoids appear to be the most significant factor in determining a species' maximum life-span potential, a logical conclusion is that individuals within the species with higher carotene levels in their tissues would be the longest lived. Tissue carotene contents can best be increased by eating and juicing a diet high in mixed carotenes.

The leading sources of carotenes are dark green leafy vegetables (such as kale, collards and spinach) and yellow-orange fruits and vegetables (such as apricots, cantaloupe, carrots, sweet potatoes, yams and squash).[14,32,33] The carotenes present in green plants are found in the chloroplasts with chlorophyll, usually in complexes with a protein or lipid. Beta-carotene is the predominant form in most green leaves, and in general, the greater the intensity of the green color, the greater the concentration of beta-carotene.

Orange colored fruits and vegetables typically have higher concentrations of provitamin A carotenes. Again, the provitamin A content parallels the intensity of the color. In the orange and yellow fruits and vegetables, beta-carotene concentrations are also high, but other carotenes are present as well, including many with more potent antioxidant and anticancer effects than beta-carotene. The red and purple vegetables and fruits (such as tomatoes, red cabbage, berries and plums) contain a large portion of nonvitamin A active pigments, including flavonoids and carotenes. Legumes, grains and seeds are also significant sources of carotenes.

Juicing provides greater benefit than beta-carotene supplements or intact carotene-rich foods because juicing ruptures cell membranes, thereby liberating important nutritional compounds like carotenes for easier absorption. The carotene found in intact foods is often poorly absorbed, and beta-carotene supplementation, while beneficial, only provides one particular type of carotene. Juicing a wide variety of carotene-rich foods will provide a broad range of carotenes, many of which have properties more advantageous than beta-carotene.[34]

You cannot consume too many carotenes. Studies done with beta-carotene have not shown it to possess any significant toxicity, even when used in very high doses in the treatment of numerous medical conditions.[3,26] However, increased carotene consumption can result in the appearance of slightly yellow to orange colored skin due to the storage of carotenes in epithelial cells. This is known as carotenodermia and is nothing to be alarmed about. In fact, it is probably a very beneficial sign. It simply indicates that the body has a good supply of carotenes.

Flavonoids
Biological Response Modifiers

The flavonoids are another group of plant pigments providing remarkable protection against free radical damage. These compounds are largely responsible for the colors of fruits and flowers. However, they serve more than aesthetic functions. In plants, flavonoids serve as protection against environmental stress. In humans, flavonoids appear to function as "biological response modifiers."

Flavonoids appear to modify the body's reactions to other compounds such as allergens, viruses and carcinogens, as evidenced by their anti-inflammatory, anti-allergic, anti-viral, and anti-carcinogenic properties.[35-37] Flavonoid molecules are quite unique in that they are active against a wide variety of oxidants and free radicals.

Recent research suggests that flavonoids may be useful in the support of many health conditions.[35-38] In fact, many of the medicinal actions of foods, juices, herbs, pollens and propolis are now known to be directly related to their flavonoid content. Over 4,000 flavonoid compounds have been characterized and classified according to chemical structure.

Different juices will provide different flavonoids and different benefits. For example, the flavonoids responsible for the red to blue colors of blueberries, blackberries, cherries, grapes, hawthorn berries and many flowers are termed *anthocyanidins* and *proanthocyanidins*. These flavonoids are found in the flesh of the fruit as well as the skin, and have very strong "vitamin P" activity.[37] Among their effects is an ability to increase vitamin C levels within our cells, decrease the leakiness and breakage of small blood vessels, protect against free radical damage, and support our joint structures.[35-37]

Flavonoids also have a very beneficial effect on collagen. Collagen is the most abundant protein of the body and is responsible for maintaining the integrity of ground substance. Ground substance is responsible for holding together the tissues of the body. Collagen is also found in tendons, ligaments and cartilage. Collagen is destroyed during inflammatory processes that occur in rheumatoid arthritis, periodontal disease, gout and other inflammatory conditions involving bones, joints, cartilage and other connective tissues. Anthocyanidins and other flavonoids affect collagen metabolism in many ways:

- They have the unique ability to cross-link collagen fibers, resulting in reinforcement of the natural collagen matrix of connective tissues.
- They prevent free radical damage with their potent antioxidant and free radical scavenging action.
- They inhibit destruction to collagen structures by enzymes secreted by our own white blood cells during inflammation.
- They prevent the release and synthesis of compounds such as histamine that promote inflammation.

These remarkable effects on collagen structures and their potent antioxidant activity make the flavonoid components of berries extremely useful in cases of arthritis and hardening of the arteries. Cherry juice has been shown to be of great benefit in gout, and feeding proanthocyanidin flavonoids from grape seeds to animals has resulted in decreases in serum cholesterol levels as well as reversal of the plaques of atherosclerosis (hardening of the arteries).[39,40] As atherosclerotic processes are still the major killers of Americans, foods rich in anthocyanidins and proanthocyanidins appear to offer significant prevention as well as a potential reversal of the process.

Still other flavonoids are remarkable anti-allergen compounds, modifying and reducing all phases of the allergic response.[35-38,41,42]

Flavonoid Content of Selected Foods

Milligrams (mg) per 100 grams edible portion (100 grams = 3.5 ounces)

Foods	4-Oxo-flavonoids[1]	Antho-cyanins	Catechins[2]	Biflavans
Fruits				
Grapefruit	50			
Grapefruit juice	20			
Oranges, Valencia	50-100			
Orange juice	20-40			
Apples	3-16	1-2	20-75	50-90
Apple juice				15
Apricots	10-18		25	
Pears	1-5		5-20	1-3
Peaches		1-12	10-20	90-120
Tomatoes	85-130			
Blueberry		130-250	10-20	
Cherries, sour		45		25
Cherries, sweet			6-7	15
Cranberries	5	60-200	20	100
Cowberries		100	25	100-150
Currants, black	20-400	130-400	15	50
Currant juice		75-100		
Grapes, red		65-140	5-30	50
Plums, yellow		2-10		
Plums, blue		10-25	200	
Raspberries, black		300-400		
Raspberries, red		30-35		
Strawberries	20-100	15-35	30-40	
Hawthorn berries			200-800	
Vegetables				
Cabbage, red		25		
Onions	100-2,000	0-25		
Parsley	1,400			
Rhubarb		200		
Miscellaneous				
Beans, dry		10-1,000		
Sage	1,000-1,500			
Tea	5-50		10-500	100-200
Wine, red	2-4	50-120	100-150	100-250

[1] 4-Oxo-flavonoids: the sum of flavanones, flavones, and flavanols (including quercetin)
[2] Catechins include proanthocyanidins

Source: Kuhnau J: The flavonoids: a class of semi-essential food components:
their role in human nutrition. *Wld Rev Nutr Diet* 24:117-91, 1976

Specifically, they inhibit the formation and secretion of potent inflammatory compounds that produce the allergic response. Several prescription medications developed for allergic conditions (such as asthma, eczema and hives) were actually patterned after flavonoid molecules. An example of an anti-allergy flavonoid is quercetin, which is available in many fruits and vegetables. Quercetin is a potent antioxidant that inhibits the release of histamine and other allergenic compounds.[34,35,40,41]

Chlorophyll
Nature's Cleansing Agent

Chlorophyll is the green pigment of plants found in the chloroplast compartment of plant cells. It is in the chloroplast where electromagnetic energy (light) is converted to chemical energy in the process known as photosynthesis. The chlorophyll molecule is essential for this reaction to occur.

The natural chlorophyll found in green plants is fat soluble. Most of the chlorophyll products found in health stores, however, contain water-soluble chlorophyll. Because water-soluble chlorophyll is not absorbed from the gastrointestinal tract, its use is limited to ulcerative conditions there.[43] Its beneficial effect is largely due to its astringent qualities and its ability to stimulate wound healing. These healing effects have also been noted with the topical administration of water-soluble chlorophyll in the treatment of skin wounds.[44] Water-soluble chlorophyll is used medically to help control body, fecal and urinary odor.[45,46]

In order to produce a water-soluble chlorophyll, the natural chlorophyll molecule must be altered chemically. The fat-soluble form, the natural form of chlorophyll as found in fresh juice, offers several advantages over water-soluble chlorophyll. This is particularly true regarding chlorophyll's ability to stimulate hemoglobin and red blood cell production, and to relieve excessive menstrual blood flow.[47,48] In fact, it is interesting to note that the chlorophyll molecule is very similar to the heme portion of the hemoglobin molecule of our red blood cells.

Heme

Portion of Hemoglobin Molecule

Chlorophyll

Unlike water-soluble chlorophyll, fat-soluble chlorophyll is absorbed very well by the rest of the body and contains other components of the chloroplast complex (including beta-carotene and vitamin K_1) that possess significant health benefits. Water-soluble chlorophyll does not provide these additional benefits.

Like the other plant pigments, chlorophyll also possesses significant antioxidant and anticancer effects.[49] It has been suggested that chlorophyll be added to certain beverages, foods, chewing tobacco and tobacco snuff to reduce cancer risk. A better recommendation would be to include fresh green vegetable juices regularly in the diet. Greens such as parsley, spinach, kale and beet tops are not only rich in chlorophyll, they are rich sources of carotenes and minerals like calcium. Parsley or some other green should be consumed along with any fried, roasted or grilled foods, as parsley has been shown to reduce the cancer-causing risk of fried foods in human studies.[50] Presumably other greens would offer similar protection.

Enzymes
Necessary for Life

Fresh juice is referred to as a "live" food because it contains active enzymes. As mentioned earlier, enzymes often work with vitamins in speeding up chemical reactions. Without enzymes there would be no life in our cells. Enzymes are far more prevalent in raw foods such as fresh juices because they are extremely sensitive to heat and are destroyed during cooking and pasteurization.

There are two major types of enzymes: synthetases and hydrolases. The synthetases help build body structures by making or synthesizing larger molecules. The synthetases are also referred to as metabolic enzymes. The hydrolases work to break down large molecules into smaller ones by adding water to the larger molecule. This process is known as hydrolysis. The hydrolases are also known as digestive enzymes.

Digestion is the body process which utilizes the greatest level of energy. That is why one of the key energy enhancing benefits of fresh juice is its highly digestible form. When you eat, your body works very hard at separating out the juice from the fiber in your food. (Remember, it is the juice that nourishes our cells.) An automatic juice extractor does this for the body, but that is not the only benefit to digestion with fresh juice. Fresh juice and other "live" foods contain digestive enzymes that help to break down the foods in the digestive tract, thereby sparing the body's valuable digestive enzymes.

This sparing action is referred to as the *Law of Adaptive Secretion of Digestive Enzymes.*[51,52] According to this law, if some of the food is digested by the enzymes contained in the food, the body will secrete less of its own enzymes. This allows vital energy in the body to be shifted from digestion to other body functions such as repair and rejuvenation. Fresh juices require very little energy to digest. In as little as five minutes, they begin to be absorbed. In contrast, a big meal of steak and potatoes may sit in the stomach for hours. If a meal is composed entirely of cooked (no enzyme) foods, most of the body's energy is directed at digestion. What happened to your energy levels after your last large meal of cooked foods? If you are like most people, your energy levels fell dramatically. What would your life be like if you directed less energy towards digestion and more energy to other body functions? It would be a life of increased energy, vitality and health.

For maximum energy levels, it is often recommended that approximately 50–75 percent of your diet (by volume) should come from raw fruits, vegetables, nuts and seeds.[53] Juicing enables you to easily reach this percentage.

Enzymes and Human Health

The best example of the beneficial effects of plant enzymes is perhaps bromelain, the enzyme found in the pineapple plant. Bromelain was introduced as a medicinal agent in 1957, and since that time, over 200 scientific papers on its therapeutic applications have appeared in the medical literature.[54,55]

Bromelain has been reported in these scientific studies to exert a wide variety of beneficial effects, including assisting in digestion; reducing inflammation in cases of arthritis, sports injury or trauma; preventing swelling (edema) after trauma or surgery; inhibiting blood platelet aggregation; enhancing antibiotic absorption; relieving sinusitis; inhibiting appetite; and enhancing wound healing.

The medical conditions for which Bromelain has proven clinically effective include:

- Angina
- Arthritis
- Athletic injury
- Bronchitis
- Burn debridement
- Cellulitis
- Dysmenorrhea
- Ecchymosis
- Edema
- Maldigestion
- Pancreatic insufficiency
- Phytobezoar
- Pneumonia
- Scleroderma
- Sinusitis
- Staphylococcal infection
- Surgical trauma
- Thrombophlebitis

Although most studies have utilized commercially prepared bromelain, it is conceivable that drinking fresh pineapple juice could exert similar, if not superior, benefits. One question that often comes up when talking about enzymes is whether or not the body actually absorbs enzymes in their active form. There is definite evidence that, in both animals and man, up to 40 percent of bromelain given by mouth is absorbed intact, without being broken down.[56-58] This provides some evidence that other plant enzymes may also be absorbed intact and exert beneficial effects as well.

Anutrients
Provide the Unknown Benefits

Fresh juice contains a wide range of substances often collectively referred to as anutrients. Included in this category are several compounds of the elements described above—carotenes, flavonoids, chlorophyll and enzymes. Nutrients are classically defined as substances that either provide nourishment or are necessary for body functions or structures. Although the designation *anutrient* signifies that these compounds are without nutritional benefit, they do exert fantastic health benefits.

Every year additional anutrients are discovered in foods that produce remarkable health-promoting effects. This emphasizes the importance of not relying on vitamin and mineral supplements alone to supply all of your nutritional needs. Vitamin and mineral supplements are designed as "supplements" to a healthy diet. A healthy diet must include not only adequate levels of known nutrients, but must also contain high quantities of fresh fruits and vegetables for their high content of "unknown" nutrients and accessory healing components.

For example, one of the American Cancer Society's key dietary recommendations to reduce the risk of cancer is to include cruciferous vegetables, such as cabbage, broccoli, Brussels sprouts and cauliflower in the diet.[5] Consumption of these foods has been shown to exert a protective effect against the development of many types of cancer that is beyond the protective effect of their known nutrient content.[4] The anti-cancer compounds in cabbage family vegetables include phenols, indoles, isothiocyanates and various sulfur-containing compounds. These compounds contain no real nutritional activity and are therefore examples of anutrients. However, these cabbage-family compounds stimulate the body to detoxify and eliminate cancer-causing chemicals.

Health Benefits of Selected Anutrients

Anutrient	Health Benefits	Food Sources
Allium compounds	Lower cholesterol levels, anti-tumor properties	Garlic and onions
Carotenes	Antioxidant, enhance immune system, anti-cancer properties	Darkly colored vegetables such as carrots, squash, spinach, kale, parsley; also cantaloupe, apricots, and citrus fruits
Coumarins	Antitumor properties, immune enhancement, stimulate antioxidant mechanisms	Carrots, celery, beets, citrus fruits
Dithiolthiones	Block the reaction of cancer-causing compounds with our cells	Cabbage-family vegetables
Flavonoids	Antioxidant, antiviral and anti-inflammatory properties	Fruits, particularly darker fruits like cherries, blueberries; also vegetables, including tomatoes, peppers, and broccoli
Glucosinolates & Indoles	Stimulate enzymes that detoxify cancer-causing compounds	Cabbage, Brussels sprouts, kale, radishes, mustard greens
Isothiocyanates &Thiocyanates	Inhibit damage to genetic material (DNA)	Cabbage-family vegetables
Limonoids	Protect against cancer	Citrus fruits
Phthalides	Stimulate detoxification enzymes	Parsley, carrots, celery
Sterols	Block the production of cancer-causing compounds	Soy products, whole grains, cucumbers, squash, cabbage-family vegetables

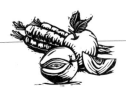

3
Juicing for a Healthy Diet & Lifestyle

Juicing is a fantastic way to improve the quality of nutrition in your diet, but juice should not be viewed as the only thing you consume. At Trillium, we support the recommendations of many medical organizations that the diet should focus on plant-based foods—vegetables, fruits, grains, legumes, nuts and seeds. In fact, we strongly support the New Four Food Groups as recommended by the Physicians Committee for Responsible Medicine. These four food groups are:

- Fruits
- Vegetables
- Whole grains
- Legumes

A diet based on the New Four Food Groups not only makes sense from a health standpoint, it makes sense from an environmental viewpoint as well. In *Diet for a New America,* John Robbins paints a graphic portrait of the consequences of the typical American eating habits on individual health, on the environment, on our natural resources and on our planet as a whole.[59] This book is essential reading for anyone concerned about the environment, their health or the earth.

The statistics opposite, excerpted from *Diet for a New America*, show clearly the impacts of a diet based on the New Four Food Groups. An increase in our consumption of fruits, vegetables, grains and legumes means a decrease in our dependence on meat and dairy products. This in turn leads to corresponding improvements in our health, environment and natural resources. Juicing provides a convenient and healthy way to incorporate such dietary changes into our everyday lives.

Incorporating Juicing as a Way of Life

Juicing is extremely easy to incorporate into your life. Simply make a habit of drinking at least 16 ounces of juice each day. Fresh juice is a great way to start off your day—it's a great substitute for that morning cup of coffee. If you work away from home, make enough juice in the morning to fill your thermos and take it to work with you. A mid-morning or mid-afternoon juice "pick-me-up" is a great way to keep your energy levels high. At lunch and dinner, start your meal with a "salad-in-a-glass." Once you start experiencing some of the benefits of juicing, it will be easy to remember the importance of fresh fruit and vegetable juices in your daily routine.

Fresh Juice vs. Whole Fruits and Vegetables

You may ask "Why Juice? Shouldn't I eat whole fruits and vegetables to get the fiber?" Of course you should, and you should juice too. Juicing fresh fruits and vegetables does provide some fiber, particularly the soluble fiber. And it is the soluble fiber that has been shown to lower cholesterol levels. Think about it—fiber refers to *indigestible* material found in plants. While this is very important for proper bowel function, it is the juice that nourishes us. Our body actually converts the food we eat into juice so that it can be absorbed. Juicing helps the body's digestive process and allows for

Effects of an Animal-Product Diet On:

Your Health

Risk of death from heart attack for average American man: **50%**

Risk of death from heart attack for American man who consumes no meat: **15%**

Increased risk of breast cancer for women who eat meat daily compared to less than once a week: **3.8 times higher**

Increased risk of fatal ovarian cancer for women who eat eggs three or more days a week compared to less than once a week: **3 times higher**

The Environment

A driving force behind the destruction of the tropical rain forests: **American meat habit**

Water pollution attributable to U.S. agriculture including runoff of soil, pesticides, and manure: **Greater than all municipal & industrial sources combined**

Our Natural Resources

Number of acres of U.S. forest that have been cleared to create cropland, pastureland, and rangeland currently producing a meat-centered diet: **260,000,000**

Number of acres of U.S. land that could be returned to forest if Americans adopted a meat-free diet and ceased exporting livestock feed: **204,000,000**

User of more than half of all water consumed for all purposes in the United States: **Livestock production**

In California, gallons of water needed to produce one edible pound of:

Tomatoes	23	Milk	130
Lettuce	23	Eggs	544
Wheat	24	Chicken	815
Carrots	33	Pork	1,630
Apples	49	Beef	5,214

Source: Robbins J: *Diet for a New America.* Stillpoint Publishing, Walpole, NH 1987. Excerpted from: *Realities for the 90s.*

quick absorption of high quality nutrition. The result? Increased energy levels. Juicing quickly provides the most easily digestible and concentrated nutritional benefits of fruits and vegetables.

Fresh Juice vs. Canned, Bottled or Frozen Juices

Fresh juice is far superior to canned, bottled or frozen juices. Fresh juice not only contains greater nutritional values, it contains life. Specifically, fresh juice contains enzymes and other "living" ingredients. In contrast, canned, bottled and packaged juices have been pasteurized. The pasteurization process keeps them on the shelf longer, but causes the loss of identifiable nutrients like vitamins and minerals, as well as the loss of other factors which are not yet fully understood.

To illustrate this, a group of researchers designed a scientific study to determine the antiviral activity of fresh vs. commercial apple juice.[32] The researchers compared the antiviral activity of fresh apple juice to commercial apple juice from concentrate, apple cider and apple wine. The results? The most potent antiviral activity was found in fresh apple juice. Why? Commercial apple juices are produced using methods like pasteurization that destroy enzymes. In doing so, a great deal of the antiviral activity is lost as well. This study clearly demonstrates the superiority of fresh juices over commercially available pasteurized juices and fruit-flavored drinks.

However, there is even more evidence to support the superiority of fresh juice. Fresh apples contain ellagic acid, glutathione and many other compounds that exert significant anticancer effects. Ellagic acid has been referred to as a "new breed of anticancer drugs." A great deal of exciting research has been done on ellagic acid. One of its primary actions is to protect against damage to our chromosomes and block the cancer-causing actions of many pollutants. Fresh whole apples and fresh apple juice contain approximately 100–130 mg per 100 grams (roughly 3½ ounces) of these valuable compounds. The content of these compounds in canned, bottled or frozen apple juice is at or near zero.

Although fresh juice is greatly superior in health benefits to processed juice products, it must be pointed out that it loses potency during storage. To get the maximum benefit from apple juice's antiviral activity, or the benefits of any other fruit or vegetable, it is best to drink the freshest juice possible.

Fresh Juice vs. Processed Food Products

There is a wide spectrum of foods—from fresh whole foods to highly processed refined food products—offered in the American food supply. An excellent illustration of this is the orange, which has evolved in the following manner:

Modern Evolution of the Orange

Raw, whole oranges or
freshly prepared orange juice

⬇

Refined, processed (pasteurized)
unsweetened orange juice

⬇

Refined, processed, sweetened
orange juice or concentrate

⬇

Refined, highly processed, sweetened,
artificially colored and flavored "orange" drinks

⬇

Completely fabricated products
never before known (such as Tang™)

At each step in this modern evolution of the orange, there is a loss of nutritional value. For example, the vitamin C content of pasteurized orange juice is extremely unreliable. Like most processed juices, the total nutritional quality is substantially lower than that of fresh orange juice. This is particularly true for juices stored in paperboard containers lined with wax or polyethylene. These products will lose up to 75 percent of their vitamin C content within three weeks.[14] Frozen juice concentrates fare no better, and orange drinks have no vitamin C unless it is added.

It should also be emphasized that in the latter stages listed above, there is not only a decrease in nutritional value, there is an increase in the number of synthetic additives. More and more food additives (like preservatives, artificial colors, artificial flavorings and acidifiers) are being shown to be extremely detrimental to our health. Although many food additives have been banned because they were found to cause cancer, there are still a great number of synthetic food additives still in use that are being linked to such diseases as depression, asthma, allergies, migraine headaches and hyperactivity or learning disabilities in children. Obviously, the ingestion of synthetic food additives needs to be avoided.

Although the government has banned many synthetic food additives, it should not be assumed that the additives currently in our food supply are safe. An example to support this is the recent (1986) ban of sulfites. Certain sulfite compounds have been used to prevent fresh fruits and vegetables from browning. Sulfites were widely used on produce at restaurant salad bars. Because most people were not aware that sulfites were being added, and because they were also unaware they had a sensitivity to sulfites, many unsuspecting people experienced severe allergic or asthmatic reactions. For years the FDA refused to consider a ban on sulfites, even while admitting that these agents provoked attacks in an unknown number of people, and in 5–10 percent of asthma victims. It was not until 1985, when sulfite sensitivity was linked to 15 deaths between 1983 and 1985, that the FDA agreed to review the matter. In 1986, the FDA finally banned sulfite use.

Clearly, the best way to reduce the need for such preservatives and other synthetic additives is to eat as many fresh and natural foods as possible. Juicing fresh fruits and vegetables is not only a great way to increase your dietary intake of important nutritional components, but helps you to avoid the majority of harmful additives and preservatives. This is especially true if you juice only organic produce.

Maintaining the Nutritional Value of Juice

Like commercial processing methods, home handling and cooking also means a loss of nutrients. For example, leafy vegetables will lose up to 87 percent of their vitamin C content upon cooking, while carrots, potatoes and other root vegetables will lose up to 33 percent for vitamin B_1, 45 percent for B_2, 61 percent for B_3 and 76 percent for vitamin C.[33] Fruits and vegetables don't have to be cooked, however, to lose nutritional value. They will also lose nutritional value if exposed to air. For example, if you slice a cantaloupe and leave the slices uncovered in the refrigerator, they will lose 35 percent of their vitamin C content within 24 hours.[33] Freshly sliced cucumbers, if left standing, will lose between 41 percent and 49 percent of their vitamin C content within the first three hours.[33] From this information we can easily conclude that it is best to drink fresh juice as soon as it is prepared. If this is not possible, juice should be stored in a thermos or in an air-tight container in the refrigerator.

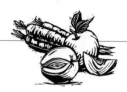

4

Juicing and Health Care

Hippocrates said, "Let your food be your medicine and let your medicine be your food." Many juices do indeed appear to have therapeutic effects, and several of these are discussed in the following pages. However, though there are specific juices that have been shown to offer benefit in certain health conditions, juices in general should not be viewed as drugs. Rather, juicing should be incorporated as a regular part of a healthy diet and lifestyle. You should also juice a wide assortment of fruits and vegetables rather than rely on any one juice to remedy a specific medical complaint. This ensures that a broad range of beneficial substances are being delivered to the body.

Juicing and Peptic Ulcers

I remember a few years ago reading the Sunday paper and noticing one of those "Ask the Doctor" type columns. The doctor was asked, "Does cabbage offer any benefit in the treatment of peptic ulcers?"

The doctor's answer was an emphatic *no*, and he went on to say that in his opinion, "the promotion of folklore is quackery." This response is most unfortunate for a number of reasons.

First of all, fresh cabbage juice has been well documented in medical literature as having remarkable success in the treatment of peptic ulcers. Dr. Garnett Cheney from Stanford University's School of Medicine, and other researchers in the 1940s and 1950s, performed several studies on fresh cabbage juice.[60,61] The results of these studies demonstrated that fresh cabbage juice is extremely effective in the treatment of peptic ulcers. In fact, the majority of patients experienced complete healing in as little as seven days. Cabbage juice works by increasing the amount of protective substances that line the intestine. A breakdown in the integrity of this lining is what causes most ulcers.

Another disturbing part of the doctor's response was his recommendation of the drugs *Tagamet* and *Zantac*. Each year, these two drugs fight it out to see which is going to be the most widely prescribed drug in the U.S. (In 1989 it was Zantac and in 1990 and 1991 it was Tagamet.) The two drugs have combined sales of over $1 billion in the U.S. alone, and $4 billion worldwide. The companies that produce these drugs consider them "perfect drugs" because they are not only expensive (a full therapeutic dose usually costs about $150 per month), they have the highest relapse rate (92 percent) of any anti-ulcer treatment. The result? A person becomes dependent on a very expensive drug because without it, the ulcer will likely come back.

Are these really perfect drugs? For most people the answer is definitely *no*. Tagamet and Zantac are associated with a number of side effects, including digestive disturbances, nutritional imbalances, liver dysfunction, disruption of bone metabolism and the development of breasts in men.[62]

The naturopathic approach to peptic ulcers is to first identify and then eliminate or reduce all factors which can contribute to the development of peptic ulcers: food allergy, cigarette smoking, stress and drugs such as aspirin and other non-steroidal analgesics. Once the causative factors have been controlled or eliminated, the focus is directed at healing the ulcers and promoting tissue resistance. This includes not only drinking cabbage juice, but eating a diet high in fiber and low in allergenic foods, avoiding those factors known to promote ulcer formation (such as smoking, alcohol, coffee and aspirin), and incorporating an effective stress reduction plan.

Juicing and Cancer

Although juicing provides benefit to nearly everyone, for one group it should be viewed as essential—people undergoing chemotherapy or radiation therapy for cancer. In addition to dealing with cancer, these individuals are subjected to a tremendous increase in their free radical load as a result of their medical treatment. They desperately need the nutritional support and protection offered by fresh fruit and vegetable juices.

Chemotherapy and radiation expose healthy cells, as well as cancer cells, to free radical damage. This results in great stress to antioxidant mechanisms and the depletion of valuable antioxidant enzymes and nutrients. Juicing provides important antioxidants and accessory nutrients that can protect against some of the damaging effects of chemotherapy and radiation.[63-65]

About two-thirds of all people with cancer develop a condition known as cachexia. Cachexia is characterized by a loss of appetite, which results in decreased nutrient intake. This in turn leads to malnutrition and muscle wasting. This is quite serious, as cachexia greatly reduces the quality of life and contributes greatly to the development of further illness or even the death of the patient. Juicing is used as part of the nutritional support program for cancer patients in several cancer treatment centers across the country.

Juicing and Arthritis

Bromelain, from fresh pineapple, was mentioned earlier as an anti-inflammatory enzyme that has been used in arthritis. Many people with arthritis may get some relief from pineapple juice, but simply drinking pineapple juice and ignoring other dietary aspects will probably not be very effective in the long run.

Diet has been strongly implicated in many forms of arthritis for several years, both in regard to cause and cure. Various practitioners have recommended all sorts of specific diets for arthritis, especially the most severe form—rheumatoid arthritis. For example, elimination of allergenic foods has been shown to offer significant benefit to some individuals with rheumatoid arthritis.[66-68] Fasting or a food allergy elimination diet followed by systematic reintroduction of foods is often an effective method of isolating offending foods. Virtually any food can result in an aggravation of rheumatoid arthritis, but the most common offending foods are wheat, corn, milk and other dairy products, beef and nightshade family foods such as tomato, potato, eggplants, peppers and tobacco.

A recent study highlights the effectiveness of juicing in the relief of rheumatoid arthritis.[69] In this thirteen-month study, conducted in Norway at the Oslo Rheumatism Hospital, two groups of patients suffering from rheumatoid arthritis were compared to determine the effect of diet on their condition. One group (the treatment group) followed a therapeutic diet and the other others (the control group) were allowed to eat as they wished. Both groups started the study by visiting a health spa for four weeks.

The treatment group began their therapeutic diet by fasting for seven to ten days and then began following a special diet. Dietary intake during the fast consisted of herbal teas, garlic, vegetable broth, a decoction of potatoes and parsley, and the juices of carrots, beets and celery. Interestingly enough, no fruit juices were allowed.

After the fast, the patients reintroduced a "new" food item every second day. If they noticed an increase in pain, stiffness, or joint swelling within 2–48 hours, this item was omitted from the diet for at least seven days before being reintroduced a second time. If the food caused a worsening of symptoms after the second time, it was omitted permanently from the diet.

The results of the study indicated that short-term fasting, followed by a vegetarian diet resulted in "a substantial reduction in disease activity" in many patients. The results indicated a therapeutic benefit beyond elimination of food allergies alone. The authors suggested that the additional improvements were due to changes in dietary fatty acids.

Fatty acids are important mediators of inflammation. Manipulation of dietary fat intake can significantly increase or decrease inflammation depending on the type of fat or oil being increased. Arachidonic acid is a fatty acid that is derived almost entirely from animal sources. It contributes greatly to the inflammatory process through its conversion to inflammatory prostaglandins and leukotrienes. Vegetarian diets are often beneficial in the treatment of inflammatory conditions like rheumatoid arthritis and asthma, presumably as a result of the decrease in the availability of arachidonic acid for conversion to inflammatory compounds.[69-71]

Rheumatoid arthritis is a prime example of a very complex "multifactorial" disease. While pineapple juice may be effective in the treatment of some people with rheumatoid arthritis, if we simply use foods or juices for their "drug-like" effects, we may not be addressing many of the underlying causes of the disease. Instead of looking for a specific juice to address a specific health condition, we should focus on adopting a diet and a lifestyle that will address the contributing factors of these diseases.

Juicing with Fresh Herbs and Spices

Supplementing your juices with medicinal herbs and spices can provide great benefit. For example, most people are aware of the many health promoting properties of garlic—including antibiotic, immune enhancing, anticancer, cholesterol lowering, blood pressure reducing and detoxification enhancing activities.[55,72,73] Fresh garlic is much more potent than cooked, dried or prepared garlic, and can be added to a number of vegetable juices to make a delicious and healthy drink. To reduce some of the undesirable effects of (such as odor), it is a good idea to place a garlic clove or two in the middle of a handful of parsley (or other green leafy vegetable), feed it through the juicer and then follow it with carrots, celery or other vegetables. This will help dilute the intense flavor and odor of garlic.

Another popular addition to juice is fresh ginger. This is a great idea if a little zest is desired or if an individual is suffering from intestinal spasms, arthritis or motion sickness.[55] Historically, the majority of complaints for which ginger was used concerned the gastrointestinal system. It is generally regarded as an excellent carminative (a substance that promotes the elimination of intestinal gas) and intestinal spasmolytic (a substance that relaxes and soothes the intestinal tract).

A clue to ginger's success in eliminating gastrointestinal distress is offered by recent double-blind studies that demonstrated ginger's effectiveness in preventing the symptoms of motion sickness, especially seasickness.[74-76] In fact, in one study, ginger was shown to be far superior to Dramamine, a drug commonly used for motion sickness.[74] Ginger reduces all symptoms associated with motion sickness including dizziness, nausea, vomiting and cold sweating.

Ginger has also been used to treat the nausea and vomiting associated with pregnancy.[55] Recently, the benefit of ginger was confirmed in hyperemesis gravidarum, the most severe form of pregnancy-related nausea and vomiting.[77] This condition usually requires hospitalization. Ginger root powder at a dose of 250 mg four times a day brought about a significant reduction in both the severity of the nausea and the number of attacks of vomiting.

Ginger has also been shown to be a very potent inhibitor of the formation of inflammatory compounds (prostaglandin and thromboxanes). This could explain why ginger has been used historically as an anti-inflammatory agent. However, ginger also has strong antioxidant activities and contains a protease (a protein-digesting enzyme) that may have similar action to bromelain on inflammation.[55]

In one clinical study, seven patients with rheumatoid arthritis, in whom conventional drugs had provided only temporary or partial relief, were treated with ginger. One patient took 50 grams per day of lightly cooked ginger while the remaining six took either 5 grams of fresh or 0.1–1 gram of powdered ginger daily. All patients reported substantial improvement, including pain relief, joint mobility and decrease in swelling and morning stiffness.[78] Ginger, like garlic, has also been shown to significantly reduce serum cholesterol levels and improve liver function.[2]

Although most scientific studies have used powdered ginger root, fresh ginger root at an equivalent dosage is believed to yield even better results as it contains active enzymes. Most studies utilized 1 gram of powdered ginger root. This would be equivalent to approximately 10 grams, or one-third ounce, of fresh ginger root. Fresh ginger root is available at most grocery stores.

The addition of ginger and garlic are great examples of medicinal herbs or spices that can be used to supplement your juice. Other examples include parsley, peppermint, capsicum (red pepper), onions and dandelion greens or root.

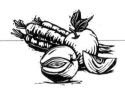

Conclusion

Thomas Edison said, "The doctor of the future will give no medicine, but will interest his patient in the care of the human frame, in diet and in the cause and prevention of disease." Unfortunately, we are still a great distance from this vision of the future. Today's health care system can better be described as a "disease care" system, in that it focuses on treating disease rather than on promoting health. Many medical organizations are realizing that the focus on looking for a cure must shift to a focus on preventing such chronic degenerative diseases as heart disease, strokes, cancer and diabetes.

Your dietary habits have a direct effect on your health, especially in the prevention of disease. That is why the first step to good health is assuming personal responsibility for it. The second step is taking the actions necessary to help you achieve the results you desire. How much is it worth to improve your health and reduce your risk of cancer, heart disease and strokes? How much is your health worth to you?

Fruits and vegetables provide numerous nutritional advantages. In their fresh form, fruits and vegetables have the greatest levels of key nutrients, and juicing is a fantastic way to significantly increase your dietary intake of these health-promoting factors. Research is showing us that it is not just the nutrients in fresh fruits and vegetables that have health-promoting properties. Equally important to good health are the anutrients like enzymes, plant pigments and various sulfur-containing compounds. Again, juicing is a phenomenal way to obtain all the healthful advantages of fresh fruits and vegetables. Don't wait until it's too late. Take action today to ensure a healthy tomorrow.

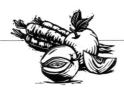

References

1   Trowell H, Burkitt D and Heaton K: *Dietary Fibre: Fibre-depleted Foods and Disease.* Academic Press, New York, NY 1985.

2   Resnicow K, Barone J, Engle A, et al: Diet and serum lipids in vegan vegetarians: a model for risk reduction. *JADA* 91:447-53, 1991.

3   Phillips RL: Role of life-style and dietary habits in risk of cancer among Seventh-Day Adventists. *Canc Res* 35:3513-22, 1975.

4   National Research Council: *Diet, Nutrition, and Cancer.* National Academy Press, Washington, DC 1982.

5   American Cancer Society. *Nutrition and Cancer: Cause and Prevention.* American Cancer Society, New York, NY 1984.

6   Wald NJ, Thompson SG, Densem JW, et al: Serum beta-carotene and subsequent risk of cancer: results from the BUPA study. *Br J Cancer* 57:428-33, 1988.

7   Harris RWC, Key TJA, Silcocks PB, et al: A case-control study of dietary carotene in men with lung cancer and in men with other epithelial cancers. *Nutr Canc* 15:63-8, 1991.

8   Peto R, Doll R, Buckley JD, et al: Can dietary beta-carotene materially reduce human cancer rates? *Nature* 290:201-8, 1981.

9   Rogers AE and Longnecker MP: Biology of disease: dietary and nutritional influences on cancer: a review of epidemiologic and experimental data. *Lab Invest* 59:729-59, 1988.

10 Ziegler RG: A review of epidemiologic evidence that carotenoids reduce the risk of cancer. *J Nutr* 119:116-22, 1989.

11 Douglass JM, Rasgon IM, Fleiss PM, et al: Effects of a raw food diet on hypertension and obesity. *South Med J* 78:841-4, 1985.

12 American Medical Association. *Drinking Water and Human Health*. American Medical Association, Chicago, IL 1984.

13 *Nutritive Value of Foods: Home and Garden Bulletin #72*. U.S. Department of Agriculture, Washington, DC 1981.

14 Shils ME and Young VR: *Modern Nutrition in Health and Disease, 7th Edition*. Lea and Febiger, Philadelphia, PA 1988.

15 Hart JP, Shearer MJ, Klenerman L, et al: Electrochemical detection of depressed circulating levels of vitamin K_1 in osteoporosis. *J Clin Endocrinol Metabol* 60:1268-9, 1985.

16 Bitensky L, Hart JP, Catterall A, et al: Circulating vitamin K levels in patients with fractures. *J Bone Joint Surg* 70-B:663-4, 1988.

17 Nielsen FH: Boron: an overlooked element of potential nutrition importance. *Nutr Today* Jan/Feb:4-7, 1988.

18 Khaw KT and Barrett-Connor E: Dietary potassium and stroke-associated mortality. *N Engl J Med* 316:235-40, 1987.

19 Jansson B: Dietary, total body, and intracellular potassium-to-sodium ratios and their influence on cancer. *Canc Det Prev* 14:563-5, 1991.

20 Iimura O, Kijima T, Kikuchi K, et al: Studies on the hypotensive effect of high potassium intake in patients with essential hypertension. *Clin Sci* 61(Suppl. 7):77S-80S, 1981.

21 Chow CK (ed): *Cellular Antioxidant Defense Mechanisms, Vols. 1–3*. CRC Press, Boca Raton, FL, 1988.

22 Fontham ETH: Protective dietary factors and lung cancer. *Int J Epid* 19(Suppl. 1):S32-S42, 1990.

23 Rosa GD, Keen CL, Leach RM and Hurley LS: Regulation of superoxide dismutase activity by dietary manganese. *J Nutr* 110:795-804, 1980.

24 Levine M: New concepts in the biology and biochemistry of ascorbic acid. *N Engl J Med* 314:892-902, 1986.

25 Burton G and Ingold K: Beta-carotene: an unusual type of antioxidant. *Sci* 224:569-73, 1984.

26 Bendich A: The safety of beta-carotene. *Nutr Cancer* 11:207-14, 1988.

27 Olson JA: 'Vitamin A,' in: Brown MB (ed): *Present Knowledge in Nutrition, 6th Edition*. Nutrition Foundation, Washington, DC 1990, pp96-107.

28 Krinsky NI: Carotenoids and cancer in animal models. *J Nutr* 119:123-6, 1989.

29 Bendich A: Carotenoids and the immune response. *J Nutr* 119:112-5, 1989.

30 Alexander M, Newmark H and Miller RG: Oral beta-carotene can increase the number of OKT4+ cells in human blood. *Immunol Letters* 9:221-4, 1985.

31 Cutler RG: Carotenoids and retinol: their possible importance in determining longevity of primate species. *Proc Natl Acad Sci* 81:7627-31, 1984.

32 Konowalchuk J and Speirs JI: Antiviral effect of apple beverages. *Appl Environ Microbiol* 36:798-801, 1978.

33 White PL and Selvey N: *Nutritional Qualities of Fresh Fruits and Vegetables*. Futura Publishing, Mount Kisco, NY 1974.

34 Bendich A and Olson JA: Biological actions of carotenoids. *FASEB J* 3:1927-32, 1989.

35   Cody V, Middleton E and Harborne JB: *Plant Flavonoids in Biology and Medicine: Biochemical, Pharmacological, and Structure-activity Relationships*. Alan R. Liss, New York, NY 1986.

36   Cody V, Middleton E, Harborne JB, and Beretz A: *Plant Flavonoids in Biology and Medicine II: Biochemical, Pharmacological, and Structure-activity Relationships*. Alan R. Liss, New York, NY, 1988.

37   Kuhnau J: The flavonoids: a class of semi-essential food components: their role in human nutrition. *Wld Rev Nutr Diet* 24:117-91, 1976.

38   Havsteen B: Flavonoids, a class of natural products of high pharmacological potency. *Biochem Pharmacol* 32:1141-8, 1983.

39   Blau LW: Cherry diet control for gout and arthritis. *Texas Rep Biol Med* 8:309-11, 1950.

40   Wegrowski J, Robert AM and Moczar M: The effect of procyanidolic oligomers on the composition of normal and hypercholesterolemic rabbit aortas. *Biochem Pharmacol* 33:3491-7, 1984.

41   Amella M, Bronner C, Briancon F, et al: Inhibition of mast cell histamine release by flavonoids and biflavonoids. *Planta Medica* 51:16-20, 1985.

42   Busse WW, Kopp DE and Middleton E: Flavonoid modulation of human neutrophil function. *J Allerg Clin Immunol* 73:801-9, 1984.

43   Rafsky HA and Krieger CI: The treatment of intestinal diseases with solutions of water-soluble chlorophyll. *Rev Gastroenterol* 15:549-53, 1945.

44   Smith L and Livingston A: Chlorophyll: An experimental study of its water soluble derivatives in wound healing. *Am J Surg* 62:358-69, 1943.

45   Nahata MC, Sleccsak CA and Kamp J: Effect of chlorophyllin on urinary odor in incontinent geriatric patients. *Drug Intel Clin Pharm* 17:732-4, 1983.

46   Young RW and Beregi JS: Use of chlorophyllin in the care of geriatric patients. *J Am Ger Soc* 28:46-7, 1980.

47   Patek A: Chlorophyll and regeneration of the blood. *Arch Int Med* 57:73-6, 1936.

48   Gubner R and Ungerleider HE: Vitamin K therapy in menorrhagia. *South Med J* 37:556-8, 1944.

49   Ong T, Whong WZ, Stewart J and Brockman HE: Chlorophyllin: a potent antimutagen against environmental and dietary complex mixtures. *Mut Research* 173:111-5, 1986.

50   Ohyama S, Kitamori S, Kawano H, et al: Ingestion of parsley inhibits the mutagenicity of male human urine following consumption of fried salmon. *Mut Research* 192:7-10, 1987.

51   Howell E: *Enzyme Nutrition*. Avery Publishing, Wayne, NJ 1985.

52   Grossman MI, Greengard H and Ivy AC: The effect of diet on pancreatic enzymes. *Am J Physiol* 138:676 82, 1943.

53   Kenton L and Kenton S: *Raw Energy*. Century Publishing, London, UK 1984.

54   Taussig S and Batkin: Bromelain: the enzyme complex of pineapple (Ananas comosus) and its clinical application: an update. *J Ethnopharmacol* 22:191-203, 1988.

55   Murray MT: *The Healing Power of Herbs*. Prima Press, Rocklin, CA 1991.

56   Miller J and Opher A: The increased proteolytic activity of human blood serum after oral administration of bromelain. *Exp Med Surg* 22:277-80, 1964.

57   Izaka K, Yamada M, Kawano T and Suyama T: Gastrointestinal absorption and

anti-inflammatory effect of bromelain. *Jap J Pharmacol* 22:519-34, 1972.

58   Seifert J, Ganser R and Brendel W: Absorption of a proteolytic enzyme of plant origin from the gastrointestinal tract into the blood and lymph of adult rats. *Z Gastroenterol* 17:1-18, 1979.

59   Robbins J: *Diet for a New America.* Stillpoint Publishing, Walpole, NH 1987.

60   Cheney G: Rapid healing of peptic ulcers in patients receiving fresh cabbage juice. *Cal Med* 70:10-14, 1949.

61   Cheney G: Anti-peptic ulcer dietary factor. *J Am Diet Assoc* 26:668-72, 1950.

62   *Physicians' Desk Reference, 45th Edition.* Medical Economics Company, Oradell, NJ 1991.

63   Sundstrom H, Korpela H, Sajanti E and Kauppila A: Supplementation with selenium, vitamin E and their combination in gynaecological cancer during cytotoxic chemotherapy. *Carcinogen* 10:273-8, 1989.

64   Hoffman FA: Micronutrient requirements of cancer patients. *Cancer* 55:295-300, 1985.

65   Judy WV, Hall JH, Dugan W, et al: 'Coenzyme Q10 reduction of adriamycin cardiotoxicity,' in: Folkers K and Yamamura Y (eds): *Biomedical and Clinical Aspects of Coenzyme Q, Vol. 4.* Elsevier Science Publications, Amsterdam, 1984, pp231-41.

66   Darlington LG, Ramsey NW and Mansfield JR: Placebo-controlled, blind study of dietary manipulation therapy in rheumatoid arthritis. *Lancet* i:236-8, 1986.

67   Hicklin JA, McEwen LM and Morgan JE: The effect of diet in rheumatoid arthritis. *Clinical Allergy* 10:463-7, 1980.

68   Panush RS: Delayed reactions to foods: food allergy and rheumatic disease. *Annals of Allergy* 56:500-3, 1986.

69   Kjeldsen-Kragh J, Haugen M, Borchgrevink CF, et al: Controlled trial of fasting and one-year vegetarian diet in rheumatoid arthritis. *Lancet* 338:899-902, 1991.

70   Ziff M: Diet in the treatment of rheumatoid arthritis. *Arthr Rheumat* 26:457-61, 1983.

71   Lindahl O, Lindwall L, Spangberg A, et al: Vegan diet regimen with reduced medication in the treatment of bronchial asthma. *J Asthma* 22:45-55, 1985.

72   Dausch JG, and Nixon DW: Garlic: A review of its relationship to malignant disease. *Preventive Med* 19:346-61, 1990.

73   Lau BH, Adetumbi MA, and Sanchez A: Allium sativum (garlic) and atherosclerosis: a review. *Nutr Res* 3:119-28, 1983.

74   Mowrey D and Clayson D: Motion sickness, ginger, and psychophysics. *Lancet* i:655-7, 1982.

75   Grontved A and Hentzer E: Vertigo-reducing effect of ginger root. *ORL* 48:282-6, 1986.

76   Grontved A, Brask T, Kambskard J and Hentzer E: Ginger root against seasickness: a controlled trial on the open sea. *Acta Otolaryngol* 105:45-9, 1988.

77   Fischer-Rasmussen W, Kjaer SK, Dahl C and Asping U: Finger treatment of hyperemesis gravidarum. *Eur J Ob Gyn Reproductive Biol* 38:19-24, 1990.

78   Srivastava KC and Mustafa T: Ginger (Zingiber officinale) and rheumatic disorders. *Med Hypothesis* 29:25-28, 1989.

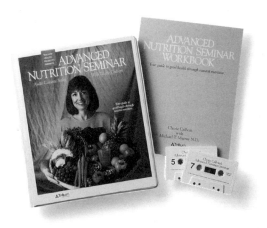

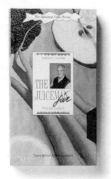
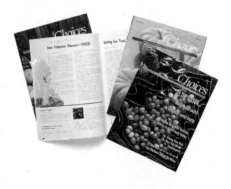